YOUR KNOWLEDGE HAS VALUE

- We will publish your bachelor's and
  master's thesis, essays and papers

- Your own eBook and book -
  sold worldwide in all relevant shops

- Earn money with each sale

Upload your text at www.GRIN.com
and publish for free

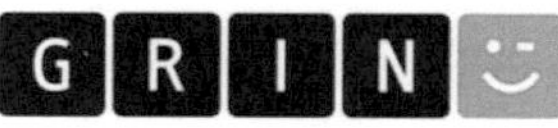

Anja Hellmann

The ethical dilemma of non-forcible Humanitarian Interventions

Utilitarian vs. Kantian Approach

GRIN Publishing

Bibliographic information published by the German National Library:

The German National Library lists this publication in the National Bibliography;
detailed bibliographic data are available on the Internet at http://dnb.dnb.de .

Imprint:

Copyright © 2010 GRIN Verlag, Open Publishing GmbH
Print and binding: Books on Demand GmbH, Norderstedt Germany
ISBN: 978-3-640-74920-1

This book at GRIN:

http://www.grin.com/en/e-book/158880/the-ethical-dilemma-of-non-forcible-
humanitarian-interventions

The ethical dilemma of non-forcible Humanitarian Interventions

Utilitarian vs. Kantian Approach

Student: Anja Hellmann

University of Southern Denmark
Campus Esbjerg
Public Health Master
Course: Critical Reflection on Public Health Research

Content

Introduction

Humanitarian Interventions (H.I.) have not only increased in the number, it has rather become a business during the past decades. Billions of Dollar are used yearly to help people all over the world. This topic deals with people, their lives and rights and is hence an extremely sensitive one. The resources must be used effective and efficient to achieve the set goals- every mistake in this way can cost lives and harm people in many ways. In my essay I will first introduce the whole field of H.I. to show the complexity and the first dilemma, which focuses on the definition of H.I., which is not consensual. Further I define and explain the topic of non- forcible H.I. The main part of this work is the analysis of the Utilitarian and the Kantian approach towards the topic of non-forcible H.I. and their critics. By the end I conclude more on a practical than on a theoretical basis- due to the fact, that the dilemmas stay as they are: dilemmas. There is no solution possible, but one can always try to find analogies in both viewpoints and start here a discussion.

1 Definition: Humanitarian Intervention

The first dilemma appears not in the actual practice of H.I., but much more already in the definition. There is no uniform definition about what H.I. is exactly about. This makes it difficult to analyze literature about this topic (Raich, 2002). Most authors define H.I. at the beginning of their essays- others don´t: Heinze (2003, p.83) e.g. sees H.I. as a "military force… for the purpose of haltering or averting human rights violations". He also cross-references to Moore, who in contrast includes the HIV- crisis in the definition for H.I. Hence, definitions differ in the include of military or non-military intervention, in the involved groups (only states or NGOs or others) and in the requirement, whether the interventions are only coercive or also consensual (Raich, 2002). In this essay I use the definition of Raich, who defines H.I. as "actions by outside parties, primarily guided by the sentiment of compassion or fellow- feeling, whose principal purpose and outcome is the alleviation of the human suffering of a foreign population without the consent of the host state" (Raich, 2002, p.21). Also Wheeler (2004) agrees, that interventions are always non-consensual and coercive- but not in general forcible. This means, that also non-military H.I. are part of it,

although those are not forcible. Further I chose to analyze the dilemmas for the non- forcibl
H.I., which can be seen in Figure 1 as Points 1,2 and 3.

Figure 1: Subgroups of Humanitarian Action

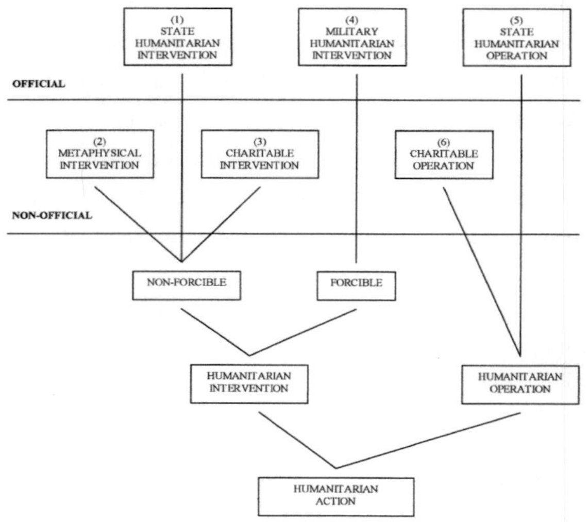

(Raich, 2004 *Ethical Evolution of the Humanitarian Idea*. p. 20)

The topic of military interventions has been frequently analyzed by many authors. The field o
the non-consent, but at the same time non-forcible measures has rarely been in focus so far
NGOs go frequently in the field, where states and other involved groups (e.g. rebels) woul
prefer them not to do so (Mills, 2005). Examples are here the intervention from the Frenc
government together with MSF[1] in Somalia, 1992 ("Rice for Somalia") (1 in figure 1), th
report from Amnesty International "China: Torture and Ill- treatment", 1996 (2 in figure1) o
the cross border interventions in Afghanistan, Laos and New Guinea, where doctors came e.g
disguised as musicians in the country, hiding their medical equipment in guitar cases (3 i
figure1) (Raich, 2004).

---

[1] MSF: Medecins sans frontieres/ Doctors without borders